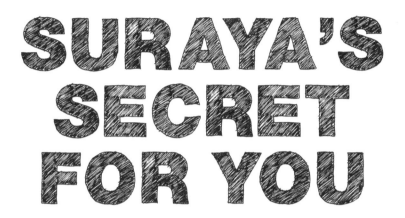

SURAYA'S SECRET FOR YOU

HOW YOU CAN CHANGE
FROM UNHAPPY TO HAPPY

DEIRDRE BROCKLEBANK (NONNA)

DISCLAIMER

FasterEFT can be fast and effective in helping to relieve stress. However, the information in this book is for educational purposes only and represents Suraya's experiences with it. Each person's experiences will vary.

SURAYA'S SECRET FOR YOU
HOW YOU CAN CHANGE FROM UNHAPPY TO HAPPY

DEDICATION

To my amazing grand-daughter Suraya who has shared her experiences of using FasterEFT (Faster Emotionally Focused Transformations) and for modelling for the photos. She is a testament to the genius of Robert G. Smith as she has benefitted from his system that seems so simple, yet it can provide profound, positive results. I hope that through Suraya's story, many children (and their parents), will be encouraged to try FasterEFT for changing their emotions and feelings, to help them to be happier and healthier.

Also to my daughter Holly, for encouraging and supporting Suraya using tapping.

WITH GRATITUDE

To Robert G. Smith whose system of FasterEFT (Faster Emotionally Focused Transformations) inspired this book. I have helped many people to change their lives through using FasterEFT. Being able to teach Robert's processes to my grandchildren has been a real bonus. This book will ensure that Robert's magic lives on in future generations, for our family and for others.

FOREWORD

This book is an easy to read guide for children and adults, about how to apply my FasterEFT tapping technique. By writing this, Deirdre is assisting me to reach my mission of helping the world one person at a time, to change their lives so they can be happier and healthier. What better place to start than with our children?

The purpose of the book is to reach children and to teach them how to change how they feel. As most of our problems develop in childhood, if they learn this simple skill it will help to make their lives easier and better as they grow up.

Robert G. Smith

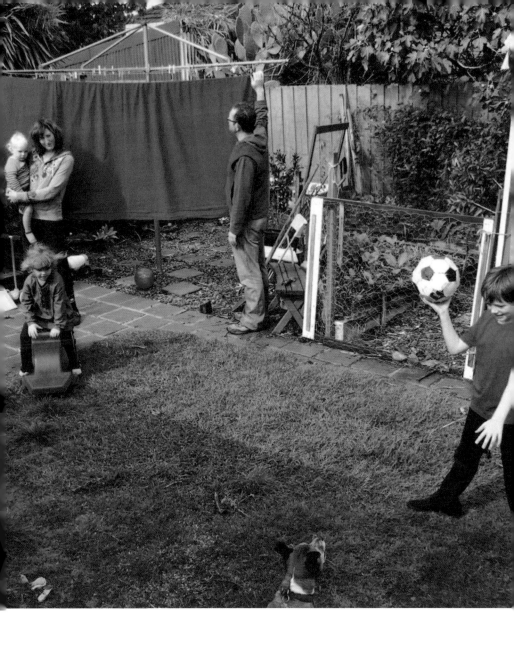

My name is Suraya. I am eight and I live in Melbourne, Australia with my mum, dad, little sister Chiara and little brother Malakai. Our dog Tia also lives with us.

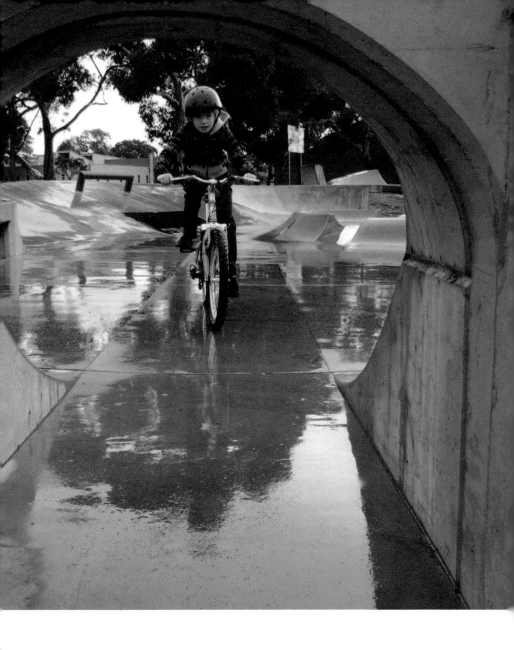

I go to the local school and I have lots of friends. I love acting, playing the keyboard and riding fast on my bike at the local park.

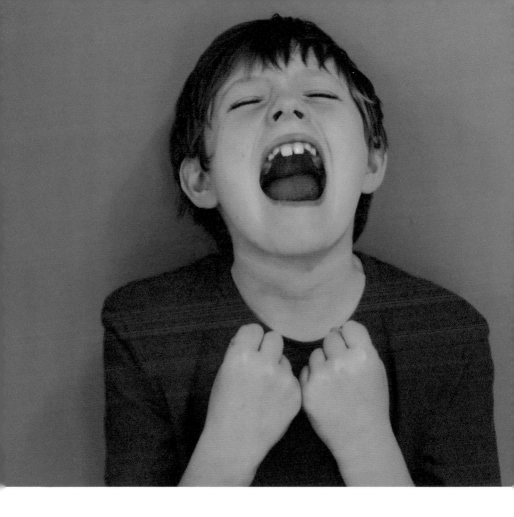

I am usually happy, but sometimes I get very angry and I yell and stamp my feet. My mum is very good and she understands that I can feel like this. I do it when I am not getting what I want or if I think something is unfair. Mum tells me that other kids may feel like this at times and we all handle things in our own way. I used to just ride my bike on my own until I felt happier. I now know another way to help me to change how I feel. Keep reading and I'll tell you about it.

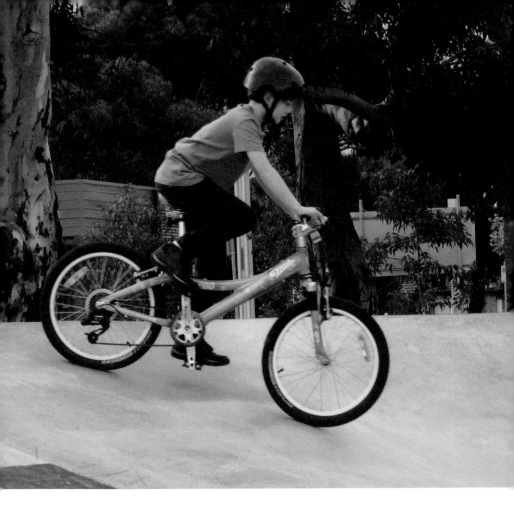

One day I fell out of the bike trailer and hurt my arm. I was shaking and my nonna said I was "in shock". I couldn't stop crying and my arm was aching. At the same time, I was remembering the time I cut my foot badly in the wheel spokes of Dad's bike. Nonna told me to notice what I felt or saw, as I thought about it. She then did something to help me feel better. She tapped on my face and the front of my chest. I was crying too much to speak so she told me to think, "I let it go" as she tapped on me and told me that it wasn't happening now.

She then held my wrist gently and told me to think of things that make me happy. I thought about all the people who love me. I started to feel better. I stopped shaking and my arm wasn't hurting as much. I was soon back on my bike again at the skate park.

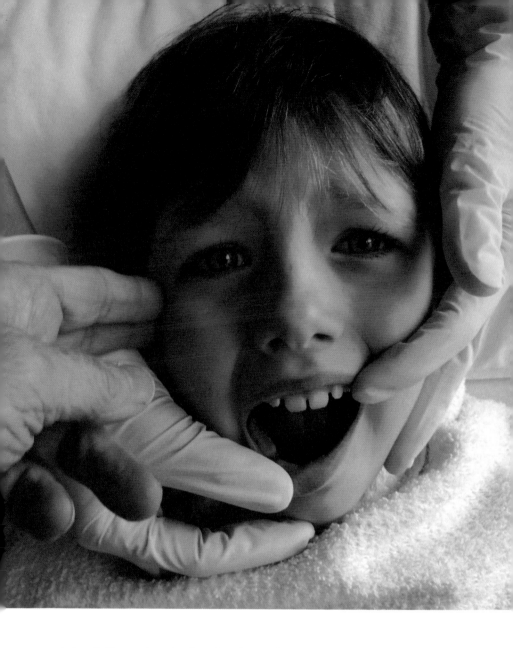

I don't like going to the dentist as it scares me. Not long ago I had to have an injection to have a tooth taken out. Nonna was with me and she helped me to relax, by tapping on me while I was in the dentist's chair. I felt calmer and less worried, especially when the dentist talked to me about Harry Potter. It was cool.

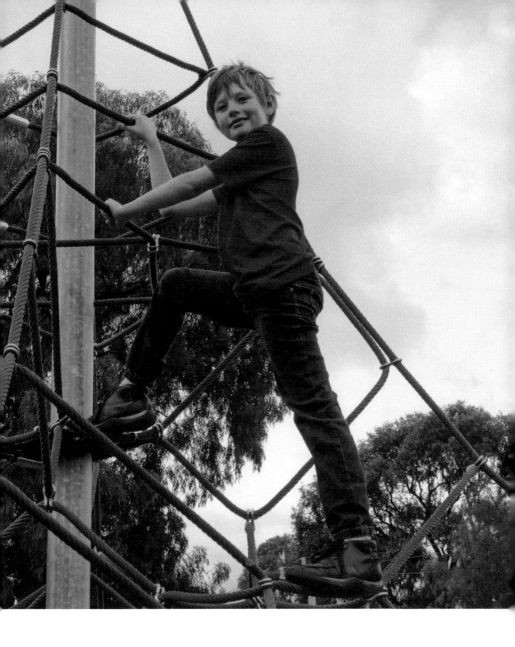

When we were driving to a park one day, I told Nonna that I felt mushy in my stomach and I felt like being sick. I tapped on myself and it went away. I felt so good that I had fun in the car and also in the park, after all!

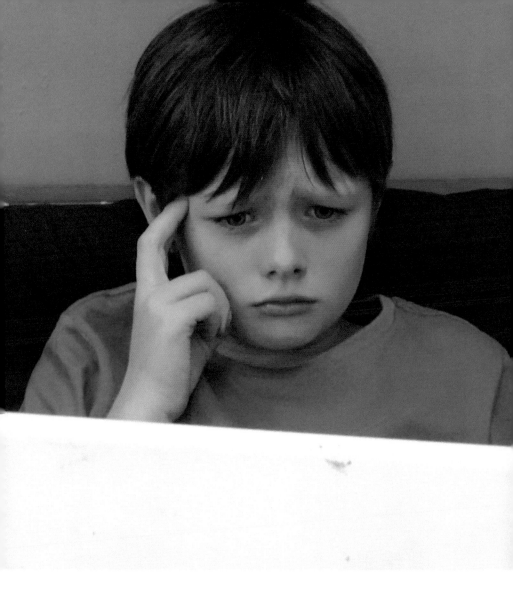

Nonna said that I can tap whenever I feel like it and to "try it on everything." I have been doing this and these are some of the other times that I have used it.

A friend told me to look at a computer game that he liked. I did look and it frightened me. Mum helped me to tap on the feeling until I felt better. I had to tap on myself again over the next few days when I thought about the game. Now I feel okay talking about it.

I was hurt at school one day, when my friend punched me in the nose. I felt sad when I thought about it later. Mum talked to me about it and she helped me to tap on what I was feeling in my body when I thought about what he did. I was a bit scared being near him at school in case it happened again. When I told Mum this, she told me that I could just imagine tapping on myself if I felt worried about it. It did happen and I did what Mum told me to do. Nobody knew I was tapping. I am not scared of him anymore.

Another day I told Nonna about a scary nightmare that I had. A big fish was eating me. As I talked about it I felt very tickly in my stomach. Nonna told me to notice how this tickly feeling felt and also to notice any pictures that I had in my mind while thinking about it. I didn't need to tap, as I just changed the picture in my head and the big fish changed into an angelfish nibbling my toes and making me laugh.

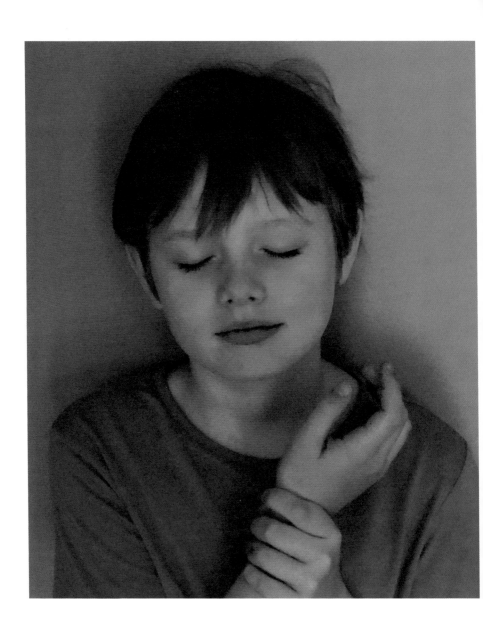

Tapping when I feel unhappy helps me to feel better. If you want to feel good too, tap along with me.

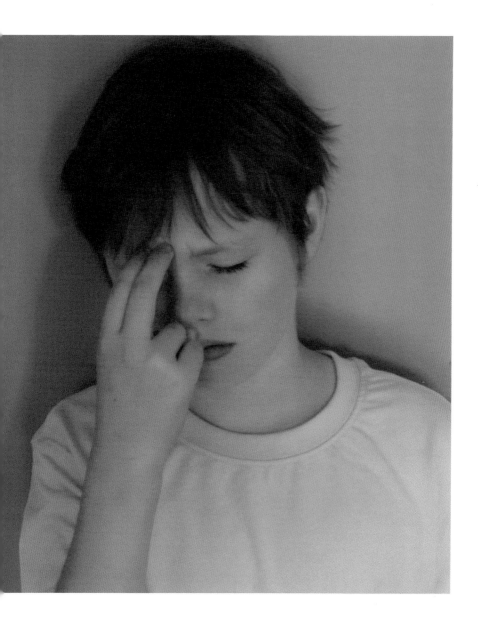

Think about what is bothering you and feel it in your body. Now tap with two fingers on the edge of your eyebrow near your nose while you think or say "I let it go."

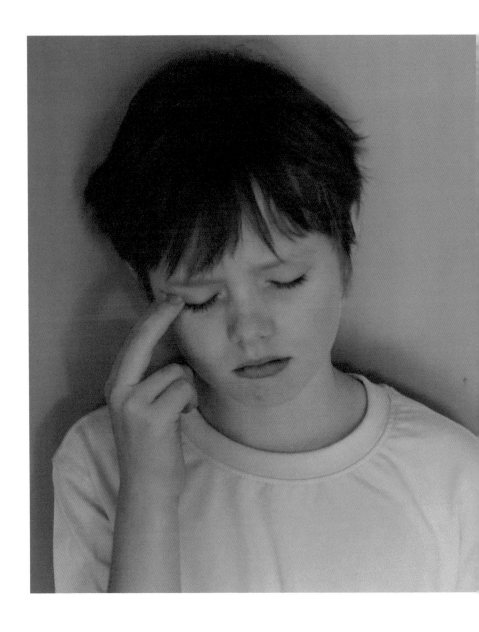

Tap next to your eye while you think or say "I let it go."

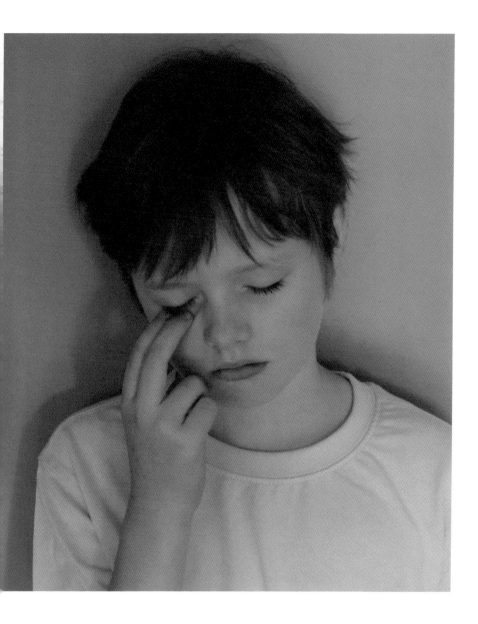

Tap in the middle under your eye while you think or say "I let it go."

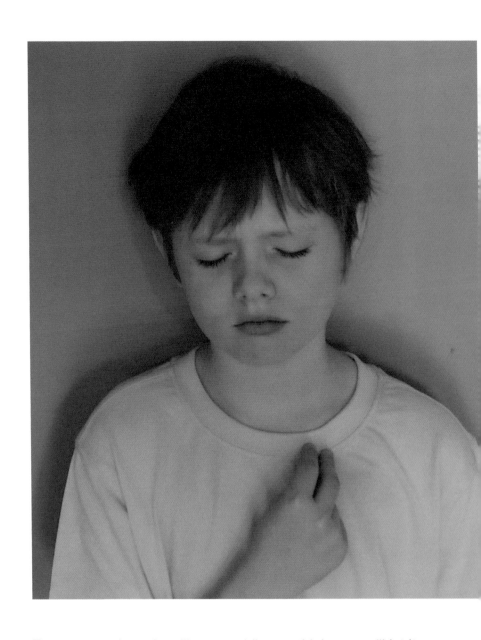

Tap on your chest, just like me, while you think or say "I let it go. It's safe to let it go."

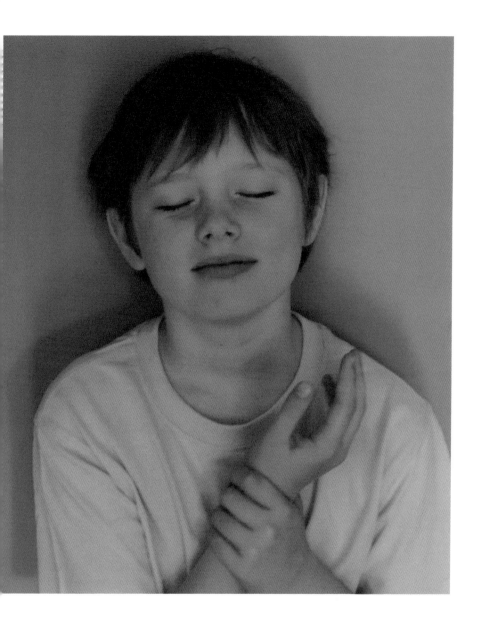

Hold around your wrist and think a happy thought. Take a deep breath, blow it out and say "Peace". Notice how much better you feel and keep tapping again from the start until you feel the best you can.

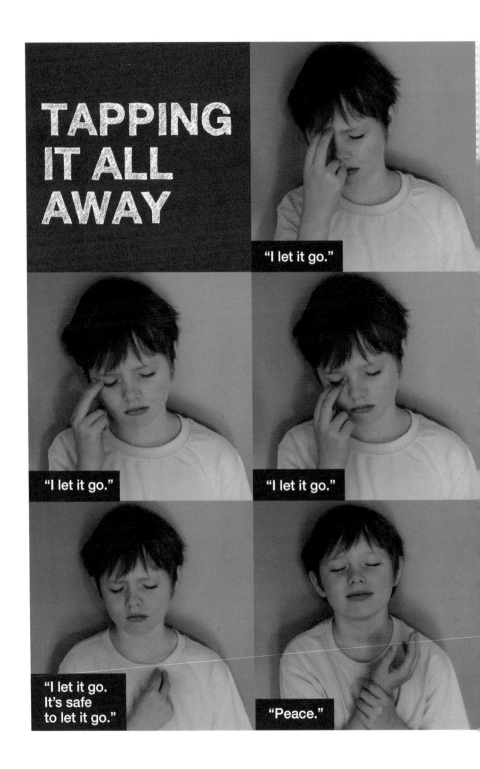

TAPPING IT ALL AWAY

"I let it go."

"I let it go."

"I let it go."

"I let it go. It's safe to let it go."

"Peace."

YOUR HAPPY LIST

(Things that make you happy)

For example, I feel happy and excited when I am at the beach. I love playing with my little brother and sister.

HOW DO YOU KNOW WHEN YOU ARE HAPPY?

- I _____

- I _____

- I _____

- I _____

- I _____

- I _____

- I _____

- I _____

- I _____

- I _____

YOUR UNHAPPY LIST

(Things to tap on)

For example, I feel sad when I have to say goodbye to people I love. I get angry when I want to watch TV and Mum says I can't.

HOW DO YOU KNOW WHEN YOU ARE UNHAPPY?

- I _____

- I _____

- I _____

- I _____

- I _____

- I _____

- I _____

- I _____

- I _____

- I _____

I help people to let go of stress so they can live happier, healthier lives.

For peace of mind – mind your peace and change how you react to a problem or issue.

For further information refer to the website for Robert G. Smith (creator of FasterEFT) www.fastereft.com and to my site www.fastereftoz.com.au

or email me at brocklebankd123@gmail.com

Scan to go directly to my site.

Deirdre Brocklebank
YOUR WELLBEING – BODY AND MIND

Printed in Great Britain
by Amazon